Tucholsky Wagner Zola Scott Sydow Freud Schlegel
Turgenev Wallace Fonatne
Twain Walther von der Vogelweide Fouqué Friedrich II. von Preußen
Weber Freiligrath Frey
Fechner Fichte Weiße Rose von Fallersleben Kant Ernst Richthofen Frommel
Hölderlin
Engels Fielding Eichendorff Tacitus Dumas
Fehrs Faber Flaubert
Eliasberg Ebner Eschenbach
Feuerbach Maximilian I. von Habsburg Fock Eliot Zweig
Ewald Vergil
Goethe London
Mendelssohn Balzac Shakespeare Elisabeth von Österreich Ganghofer
Lichtenberg Rathenau Dostojewski
Trackl Stevenson Doyle Gjellerup
Mommsen Tolstoi Hambruch
Thoma Lenz Hanrieder Droste-Hülshoff
Dach Verne von Arnim Hägele Hauff Humboldt
Karrillon Reuter Rousseau Hagen Hauptmann Gautier
Garschin
Damaschke Defoe Hebbel Baudelaire
Descartes
Hegel Kussmaul Herder
Wolfram von Eschenbach Darwin Dickens Schopenhauer Rilke George
Bronner Melville Grimm Jerome Bebel
Campe Horváth Aristoteles Barlach Federer Proust
Bismarck Vigny Voltaire Herodot
Gengenbach Heine
Storm Casanova Tersteegen Grillparzer Georgy
Chamberlain Lessing Langbein Gilm
Brentano Gryphius
Claudius Schiller Lafontaine
Strachwitz Bellamy Schilling Kralik Iffland Sokrates
Katharina II. von Rußland Gerstäcker Raabe Gibbon Tschechow
Löns Hesse Hoffmann Gogol Wilde Gleim Vulpius
Luther Heym Hofmannsthal Klee Hölty Morgenstern
Roth Heyse Klopstock Kleist Goedicke
Luxemburg Puschkin Homer Mörike Musil
La Roche Horaz
Machiavelli Kierkegaard Kraft Kraus
Navarra Aurel Musset Kind Moltke
Nestroy Marie de France Lamprecht Kirchhoff Hugo
Nietzsche Nansen Laotse Ipsen Liebknecht
Marx Ringelnatz
von Ossietzky Lassalle Gorki Klett Leibniz
May vom Stein Lawrence Irving
Petalozzi Platon Knigge
Pückler Michelangelo Kock Kafka
Sachs Poe Liebermann Korolenko
de Sade Praetorius Mistral Zetkin

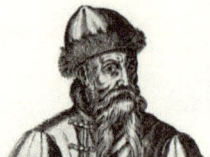

The publishing house tredition has created the series **TREDITION CLASSICS**. It contains classical literature works from over two thousand years. Most of these titles have been out of print and off the bookstore shelves for decades.

The book series is intended to preserve the cultural legacy and to promote the timeless works of classical literature. As a reader of a **TREDITION CLASSICS** book, the reader supports the mission to save many of the amazing works of world literature from oblivion.

The symbol of **TREDITION CLASSICS** is Johannes Gutenberg (1400 – 1468), the inventor of movable type printing.

With the series, tredition intends to make thousands of international literature classics available in printed format again – worldwide.

All books are available at book retailers worldwide in paperback and in hardcover. For more information please visit: www.tredition.com

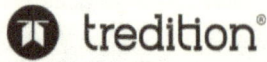

tredition was established in 2006 by Sandra Latusseck and Soenke Schulz. Based in Hamburg, Germany, tredition offers publishing solutions to authors and publishing houses, combined with worldwide distribution of printed and digital book content. tredition is uniquely positioned to enable authors and publishing houses to create books on their own terms and without conventional manufacturing risks.

For more information please visit: www.tredition.com

A Dissertation on the Medical Properties and Injurious Effects of the Habitual Use of Tobacco

A. (Alvan) McAllister

Imprint

This book is part of the TREDITION CLASSICS series.

Author: A. (Alvan) McAllister
Cover design: toepferschumann, Berlin (Germany)

Publisher: tredition GmbH, Hamburg (Germany)
ISBN: 978-3-8491-8405-6

www.tredition.com
www.tredition.de

Copyright:
The content of this book is sourced from the public domain.

The intention of the TREDITION CLASSICS series is to make world literature in the public domain available in printed format. Literary enthusiasts and organizations worldwide have scanned and digitally edited the original texts. tredition has subsequently formatted and redesigned the content into a modern reading layout. Therefore, we cannot guarantee the exact reproduction of the original format of a particular historic edition. Please also note that no modifications have been made to the spelling, therefore it may differ from the orthography used today.

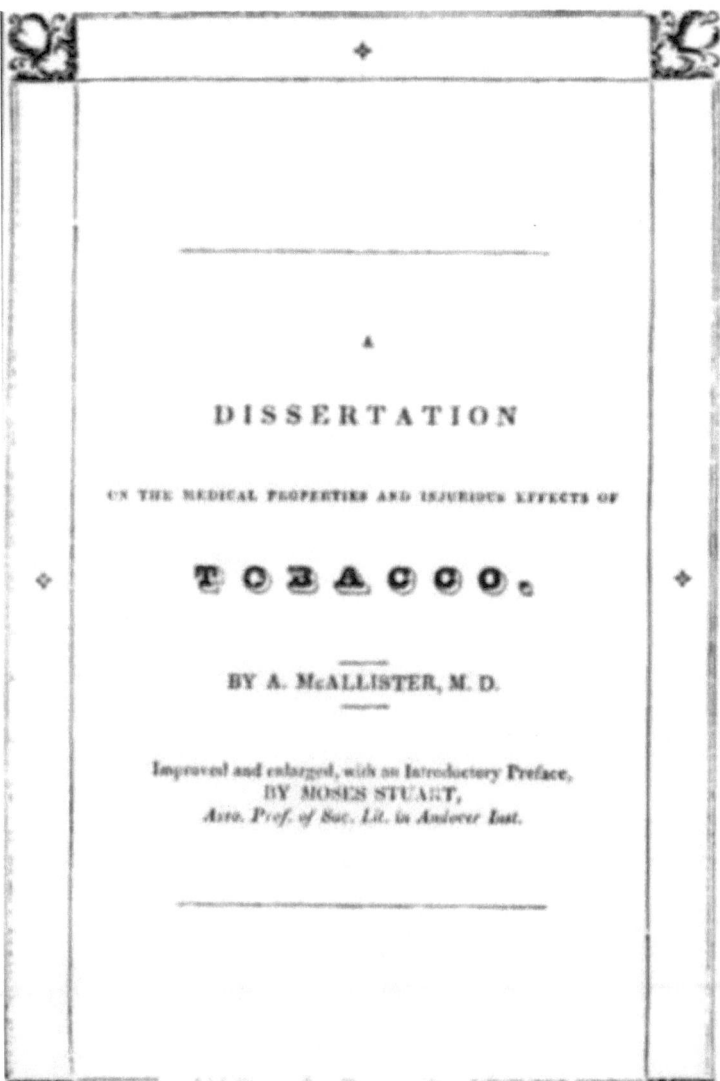

A

DISSERTATION

ON THE MEDICAL PROPERTIES AND INJURIOUS EFFECTS OF

TOBACCO.

BY A. McALLISTER, M. D.

Improved and enlarged, with an Introductory Preface,
BY MOSES STUART,
Asso. Prof. of Sac. Lit. in Andover Inst.

A DISSERTATION
ON THE
MEDICAL PROPERTIES AND INJURIOUS EFFECTS
OF THE
HABITUAL USE OF TOBACCO:

READ, ACCORDING TO APPOINTMENT, BEFORE THE MEDICAL
SOCIETY OF THE COUNTY OF ONEIDA, AT THEIR
SEMI-ANNUAL MEETING,

JANUARY 5, 1830.

BY

A. McALLISTER, M. D.

Second Edition.
Improved and enlarged, with an Introductory Preface,
BY MOSES STUART,
Associate Professor of Sac. Lit. in the Theol. Inst. at Andover.
BOSTON:
PUBLISHED BY PEIRCE & PARKER,
No. 9. Cornhill.
NEW YORK:—H. C. SLEIGHT,
Clinton Hall.

1832.

Entered, according to Act of Congress, in the year 1832, by
Peirce & Parker, in the Clerk's Office of the District Court of Massachusetts.
PRESS OF PEIRCE & PARKER.
No. 9, Cornhill.

INTRODUCTION.

The first edition of Dr. McAllister's Essay, was printed without any Appendix. Having myself been in the habit of using tobacco very moderately (usually but once in a day) from early life, I read the Essay as first printed with great interest. It appeared to me a sober, judicious, rational appeal to the understanding and judgment of the public, with respect to the subject of which it treats. A highly respected friend of mine desired me to give him my opinion of the Essay in writing. I consented to do this; and when I had done it, he judged it expedient to publish that opinion; to which I gave my consent. It was published in the *Journal of Humanity*; and for substance it was made up of an abridgement of Dr. McAllister's views, and some strictures on his style and method of treating the subject. In particular, a desire was expressed that Dr. McA. would discuss more fully some of the arguments employed in defence of using tobacco. This critique was sent to the author of the Essay; who in consequence of it expressed a willingness to revise his work, and make such additions as had been suggested. Some weeks since he transmitted to me a copy of the original edition, with a manuscript containing the Appendix to the present edition. At the same time he requested me to make any alterations in either part, which I might deem expedient. I have used this liberty so far as to change a few *technical* words for popular and intelligible ones. In some of these cases, I have detracted from the *specific* accuracy of the writer, as a medical man, for the sake of making his expressions more intelligible to the mass of readers. What he will thus lose, in his reputation for scientific accuracy, he will gain by becoming more useful. A few other slight alterations and modifications have been made; but only such as I judged the worthy author would at once cheerfully admit. I have kept within the bounds of the liberty which he gave me; and I trust he will not be dissatisfied with what I have done.

I command the serious perusal of the following Essay and Appendix to every man, who wishes to become well informed respecting the properties of tobacco. Whoever uses this substance as a luxury, is bound by a due regard to his own physical welfare to make himself acquainted with its properties and their influence. If any man can soberly peruse the following pages, without conviction that he is "playing with edge-tools," while he is indulging in the use of tobacco, I must confess his mind to be of a composition different from mine.

One word as to *breaking off the habit*. The difficulty, I fully believe, is not much less than the breaking off from ardent spirits. But as to any danger to health in breaking off, the fear is idle; excepting [i] in case of delicate habits, where small changes produce great effects; or in case of advanced years and inveterate habit, where the course of those fluids which are so much affected by tobacco, if suddenly and entirely changed, may give rise to serious inconvenience. My belief, however, is, *that there no case in which a judicious and proper course may not effect an entire weaning from the use of tobacco*. Most persons in good health, and all in younger life, may break off at once, without the least danger. Two or three days will overcome all difficulty. Those whom slight changes in regimen affect very much, may break off more gradually; and so of persons advanced in life. A good way of accomplishing this, is to procure some of the most detestable tobacco which can be found, and when appetite will not forego the use of it without an evil greater than to use it, then take it in such a quantity as will be sure to nauseate and prostrate. This will put the next dose farther off; and two or three doses thus administered, will so blunt the appetite, that quitting the practice will appear to be quite a moderate degree of self-denial. Those who never felt the appetite may laugh at such directions as these; but those who know its power, will at least think them worth some consideration.

I do not place the use of tobacco in the same scale with that of ardent spirits. It does not make men maniacs and demons. But that it does undermine the health of thousands; that it creates a nervous irritability, and thus operates on the temper and moral character of men; that it often creates a thirst for spirituous liquors; that it allures to clubs, and grog-shops, and taverns, and thus helps to make idlers and spendthrifts; and finally, that it is a very serious and needless expense; are things which cannot be denied by any observing and considerate person. And if all this be true, how can the habitual use of tobacco, as a mere luxury, be defended by anyone who wishes well to his fellow-men, or has a proper regard to his own usefulness?

I have been in the use of it for thirty-five years; but I confess myself unable, on any ground, to defend or to excuse the practice. The wants which are altogether artificial, are such as duty calls us to avoid. The indulgence of them can in no way promote our good or our real comfort.

I commend, therefore, the following sheets to the public: hoping that all, and especially the young, will read and well consider the suggestions they offer.

M. STUART.

Andover, Jan. 10, 1832.

To the Medical Society of the County of Oneida.

Gentlemen,

We have accidentally seen the manuscript copy of an address pronounced lately before your society, by Dr. McAllister. The research on which it is founded, and its perspicuity and arrangement, entitle it to a form more permanent than manuscript. But if the results are true, which it attempts to substantiate, they present imperious considerations for the publication of the address.

We are not disposed to contract the circle of enjoyment; but if mischief crouches under the covert of any pleasure, propriety requires a notification to the unwary. Even should experience warrant the conclusion that habit enables us to use tobacco with physical impunity, (a conclusion Dr. McAllister powerfully controverts,) we must concede, that its use is disgusting to persons not infected with the habit.

Civilization is composed of innumerable acts of self-denial; while the gratification of appetites, regardless of others, is the strongest feature of barbarism. We see then, even as a dictate of refinement, that the use of tobacco should be abandoned; and it has been abandoned by all the polite circles of Europe.

But tobacco possesses that strong characteristic of a bad habit; it seldom leaves its votaries the liberty of abandonment. All which the address can effect, is an admonition to youth, over whom tobacco has not yet acquired its bad supremacy. As parents, then, anxious to see our children uncontaminated by disgustful practices; as citizens, emulous that our country shall not be surpassed in refinement by the nations of Europe, we are solicitous that the address of Dr. McAllister should be published, and in a pamphlet form, under the authority of your society.

We are aware that this request involves a departure from your general disposition of the periodical addresses of your members, but we beg to suggest that the general interest of the present production renders a departure from your usual course not invidious, but a duty which we humbly think you owe to philanthropy. In support of our opinion, we take the liberty of enclosing you a letter from a distinguished fellow-citizen in Albany, who also accidentally saw the address: and we are, Gentlemen,

With very great respect, your ob't serv'ts,

A. B. JOHNSON,
D. C. LANSING,
HIRAM DENIO,
R. R. LANSING,
EDM'D A. WETMORE,
WILLIAM WILLIAMS,
SAM'L D. DAKIN.

Utica, Feb. 27, 1830.

[iii]

Lydius Street, Albany, }
Friday Evening, January 22d, 1830. }

Dear Sir,

I have just completed an attentive perusal of the manuscript *discourse on tobacco*, which you handed to me this afternoon; and I really feel obliged to the author for the interest and instruction which it has afforded me. I am sincerely of opinion that the respectable society before whom it was delivered, owe it to themselves, to the public, and to the author, (if they have not already done so,) to request its publication. And, favorably as it leads me to think of the author's intellectual and professional endowments, he must be still more distinguished for his *modesty*, if he declines a compliance with such a request. He has treated a highly important subject, in a clear, forcible, and striking manner; and the public are deeply concerned in knowing what he has said of it. I will only add, that in point of literary execution, it is, in my judgment, most decidedly respectable, and would in that respect reflect no discredit upon any medical gentleman in this state.

Very respectfully and truly yours, &c. &c.

A. CONKLING.

R. R. Lansing, Esq.

At a meeting of the Medical Society of the County of Oneida, on the 5th of March, 1830, a communication was received, signed by a number of highly respectable gentlemen from this and other counties of this state, on the subject of a dissertation delivered before this society, at their late semi-annual meeting, by Dr. McAllister, "on the properties and effects of tobacco." The communication was referred to a committee.

The committee reported, "That although dissertations so delivered became the properly of the society, yet believing as we do, that the subject is one of great importance, and the dissertation highly meritorious, and as we have not funds to defray the expense of publication, we will cheerfully relinquish our claim thereto in favor of our correspondents, and cordially unite with them in the desire which they have expressed to us, 'that the dissertation be published in a pamphlet form,' for their gratification and the benefit of the public."

Resolved, That the above report be accepted, and that a copy of the proceedings be delivered to the gentlemen who presented the communication.

C. B. COVENTRY, Sec'y pro. tem.

[iv]

PREFACE.

In consenting to the publication of the following pages, the author yielded to the request of gentlemen whose opinions he did not feel at liberty to disregard; he therefore hopes to avoid the imputation of vanity, with which he might have been charged, had he obtruded himself on the attention of the public, unsolicited. That the habitual use of tobacco is a wide spread, and spreading evil, will be acknowledged by all. This has been felt for years by the most enlightened members of the Faculty. That it causes many diseases, particularly visceral obstructions, and renders many others exceedingly difficult to cure, is demonstrated in the daily experience of every practitioner. The conviction that this habit was constantly extending by the advice and example of physicians, first induced the author to undertake the discussion of this subject before the respectable Society to which he has the honor to belong. Whether the attempt has been successful, the public will judge. That it is imperfect, will not be denied; but it is believed to have claims as a candid statement of facts.

To literary distinction the author makes no pretentions; he therefore craves the indulgence of the learned, as they can best appreciate the labor of writing well. He has chosen a free, popular style, believing that the best calculated to do good; and to render it still more familiar, at the suggestion of some friends, the technical terms have been mostly expunged. Aware that affectation consists no less in studiously avoiding, than in unnecessarily using technical language, the author submitted to this, in the hope of being better understood by persons out of the Profession. His medical brethren will, therefore, know how to excuse him, for attempting to make this essay more plain, though it should be at the expense of technical accuracy.

[v]

Should the prevalence of the practice, be a fair index to public sentiment, the author is aware that he wars against a fearful odds. But many who use this noxious weed, without hesitation acknowledge its deleterious effects, and urge in extenuation the inveteracy of habit.

One consideration had considerable influence to induce the author to consent to the publication of this paper—the hope that it might aid in putting away the evil of intemperance, by pointing out one grand source of that desolating scourge. When public attention shall be fully awakened to this subject, innumerable instances will be found, where drunkenness has followed as the legitimate consequence of using tobacco.

Should that hope be fulfilled—should it be found that the labor of the author has exerted any salutary influence, in restraining young men from falling into those habits which are inevitably followed by much physical suffering, if not by absolute ruin, such a result would be to him an ample compensation.

Utica, May, 1830.

[9]

DISSERTATION.

Mr. President and Gentlemen:

The confidence of an enlightened community has assigned to you, as guardians of the dearest interests of society, an elevated and highly responsible rank among those who labor to promote the great cause of human happiness. Your influence in the medical councils of this great and flourishing State, gives a lasting effect to your deliberations, and stamps a value on those productions which you are pleased to approve. While the opinions of other men are often exhibited and forgotten with the occasion which gave them birth, those of the physician continue not unfrequently to affect at least the physical welfare of the world, after his "dust has returned to the earth as it was, and his spirit has gone to God who gave it." In view of this momentous truth, an humble attempt will now be made, in discharge of the duty assigned me, to examine the cause of some of the "ills which flesh is heir to."

I regard this principle as an axiom, that whatever conduces to augment the sum of human happiness, must be an object of solicitude to the conscientious and intelligent physician. He will be anxious that his fellow citizens should be sober, peaceable, and virtuous; that they should be industrious, frugal, and prosperous. Whatever will produce such results should receive the decided approbation of every benevolent member of the Faculty. It follows, of course, that whatever has an opposite tendency should meet his frown. Pursuing this principle, you have condemned the use of ardent spirits, unless sickness demands their application as a medicine.

The physical evils resulting from intemperance were eloquently exhibited in the address, presented by your committee, during the last year. That address, with its accom [10] panying resolutions, now exerts a beneficial influence through a widely extended community. We are cheered by the kind wishes and prayers of the friends of good order, in our efforts to destroy that vice which has not only "walked" through our country "in darkness," but "wasted at noon-day." But while we exult in the triumph of correct principles on *this* subject, do not other vicious indulgences demand our attention? Should we slumber over the mischiefs resulting from such indulgences, while the public look to us as pioneers who should trace out the pathway to health and happiness, and demand from us both precepts and examples of sobriety and virtue? Unfortunately, in all our attempts to abolish practices prejudicial to the best interests of man, we are compelled, in the outset, to encounter our own inveterate habits—habits which rise up in mutiny against reformation, and with clamorous note forbid us to proceed. Are we so fortunate as to be free from their influence ourselves, we look around and see our friends bound in chains, from which we should rejoice to deliver them; but we fear, perhaps, to make an experiment which may rouse their passions, rather than convince their understandings.

Who can count the multitudes yearly consigned to the tomb, by the indulgence of a fastidious and unnatural appetite? Headaches, flatulencies, cholics, dyspepsias, palsies, apoplexies, and death, pursue the Epicurean train, as ravens follow the march of an armed host, to prey on those who fall in the "battle of the warrior, with their garments rolled in blood." The truth of this statement will not be questioned. Yet where is the physician, possessing sufficient moral courage to raise his voice against the system of modern cookery? Should it be thought, that, as medical men have given no more encouragement to that system than any other class in society, they are not bound to use any extraordinary exertions to produce a change; still a wide field is left open to benevolent action in reference to those things, the influence of which is injurious to mankind.

Gentlemen—there is a baneful habit, diffused, like the atmosphere, through all classes, and affecting all the ramifications of society. And this habit owes much of its prevalence to the advice and example of respectable physicians. We indulge the hope, from the great increase of medical knowledge, that the time will soon arrive, when persons disposed to vicious indulgence will be unable to entrench [11] themselves behind our professional advice. I am aware that I tread on dangerous ground, in attempting to investigate the propriety of a practice which has been introduced and approved by a large portion of the members of this respectable Society. You may start at the suggestion, and regard it as unworthy of your notice. Let me hope, however, that you will suspend your opinions, while I endeavor to present the *natural history, chemical composition,* and *medical properties* of one of our most deadly narcotics—the *Tabaci Folia, Nicotiana Tabacum,* i. e. tobacco. If in the prosecution of this inquiry, we shall be able to discover the great and injurious effects which the use of this poisonous plant produces on the constitution, I shall be excused, if I urge this subject on your consideration with more than ordinary importunity.

I. Natural History.

"This plant was unknown in Europe until after the discovery of America by the Spaniards, and was first carried to England by Sir Francis Drake, A. D. 1560. The natives of this continent call it *petun*; those of the islands, *yoli*. The Spaniards, who gave it the name of *tobacco*, took that name from Tabaco, a province in Yucatan, where they first found it, and first learned its use. Some contend that it derives its name from Tobago, one of the Caribbee Islands, discovered by Columbus, in 1498." [A] It received the name *tobacco* from Hernandez de Toledo, who first sent it to Spain and Portugal.

The botanic description of this plant may be found in most works on the science of botany: and therefore I shall not detain you with it at this time. The plant, while growing exhibits a very beautiful appearance, but is so extremely nauseous, that in all the variety of insects, only one is found to feed upon it. This is a worm "*sui generis*," the mode of its propagation being entirely unknown; and from its being the only living creature (man excepted) that will devour this plant, [B] it is called "*tobacco worm.*"

II. Sensible Qualities.

It is of a yellowish green color; it has a strong, narcotic, and fœtid odor, with a bitter and extremely acrid taste.

[12]

III. Chemical Composition.

"Mucilage, albumen, or gluten, extractive, a bitter principle, an essential oil, nitrate of potass, which occasions its deflagration, muriate of potass, and a peculiar proximate principle, upon which the virtues of the plant are supposed to depend, and which has therefore been named *Nicotin*. This peculiar principle is considered by some, as approaching the essential oil in its properties. It is colorless, has an acrid taste, and the peculiar smell of tobacco; and occasions violent sneezing. With alcohol and water it forms a colorless solution, from which it is precipitated by a tincture of galls. Tobacco yields its active matter to water and proof spirit, but most perfectly to the latter; long boiling weakens its powers. A most powerful oil may be obtained by distillation, and separating it from the surface of the water on which it floats."

IV. Medical Properties.

These are considered to be those of a powerful *narcotic, antispasmodic, emetic, cathartic, sudorific,* and *diuretic*.

"As a *narcotic*, it is endued with the most energetic, poisonous properties, producing, when administered even in small doses, severe nausea and vomiting, cold sweats, universal tremors, with extreme muscular debility." From its exerting a peculiar action on the nervous system, as ascertained by the well directed experiments of Mr. Brodie, it powerfully controls the action of the heart and arteries, producing invariably a weak, tremulous pulse, with all the apparent symptoms of approaching death. And so different is its operation from that of other narcotics, that it actually operates with more destructive efficacy, when used by way of injection, than when applied either to the skin, or when taken into the stomach.

From what has been said of its narcotic powers, you, Gentlemen, will readily infer its virtue as an article of *medicine*. If we wish, at any time, to prostrate the powers of life in the most sudden and awful manner, we have but to administer a dose of tobacco, and our object is accomplished. Hence its use in obstinate constipation, in cholic, in the iliac passion, and in stranguary.

As it is conceded that its efficacy as an *antispasmodic* [13] depends upon its power to prostrate every vestige of tone and elasticity in the muscular fibre, prudence would dictate that it should be used with the utmost circumspection, when the system had been previously exhausted by the disease, or by the antecedent method of cure. Melancholy instances are on record, of the fatal effects of this medicine when administered without this caution, both as an internal remedy, and as an external application in cutaneous diseases. Two instances will suffice.

"A medical practitioner," says Paris, "after repeated trials to reduce a strangulated hernia, injected an infusion of tobacco, and shortly after sent the patient in a carriage to the Westminster Hospital, for the purpose of undergoing the operation; but the unfortunate man arrived only a few minutes before he expired."

"I knew a woman," says the same learned author, "who applied to the heads of three of her children, afflicted with scald-head, an ointment composed of snuff and butter; but what was the poor woman's surprise, to find them immediately seized with vertigo, violent vomiting, fainting, and convulsions."

We next come to its effects as an *emetic*. "As such," says Professor Chapman, "tobacco claims our attention. Cullen and many others opposed its use, on account of the harshness of its operation. Certainly it exceeds all others in the promptness, violence, and permanence of its impressions. But these very qualities, unpleasant as they are, enhance its value in many cases."

"Tobacco seems especially to be adapted to the evacuation of some poisons; and it has this advantage, that it acts with equal certainty and expedition, when applied to the region of the stomach in the form of a poultice, as when internally administered." Professor Barton says, he had recourse to an application of the moistened leaves of this plant to the region of the stomach, with complete success, to expel an inordinate quantity of laudanum, in a case where the most active emetics, in the largest doses, were resorted to in vain. But most poisons, particularly the corrosive, are attended with so much exhaustion, that it would seem perilous to administer tobacco, lest by its own depressing effects, the powers of vitality might be irrecoverably extinguished. In many instances, however, it appears that it [14] may be administered in small doses with safety and advantage.

We are informed by a respectable writer, that while at the Cape of Good Hope, he had a number of Hottentots, with intermittent fever, under his care. Having few medicines, he resorted to tobacco, and found six grains of snuff as effectual in exciting vomiting, as two of Tartar emetic.

By many it is preferred in minute doses, as a nauseating medicine. Thus administered, it has succeeded in subduing some of the most violent symptoms of the most furious cases of mania; and where it cannot be given by the mouth, from the obstinacy of the patient, it may with equal benefit be applied in the form of a poultice.

As a *cathartic*, tobacco is entitled to notice. "Some physicians have been in the habit of prescribing this powerful substance not only for the more dangerous cases of incarcerated hernia, but in all cases of obstinate constipation, from whatever cause produced. To relieve these painful diseases, it has been usually given in the form of a clyster, regulating the dose to the age, circumstances, and strength of the patient; and it is affirmed to have proved, in many instances, very effectual, and to possess the confidence of practitioners."

I was informed by a learned and ingenious friend, that, having an obstinate case of ascaris lumbricoides in his own family, after repeated unsuccessful efforts to dislodge the worms, he at last had recourse to this potent remedy, a poultice of which he applied to the region of the stomach. The worms were almost instantaneously expelled, but with very alarming symptoms, and a complete prostration of the patient. From these circumstances, we should be led to conclude, that its efficacy as a vermifuge defends either upon its narcotic properties, or upon its sudden and powerful effect as a cathartic.

Its effects as a *sternutatory*, i. e. as exciting to sneeze, are known to all. If applied to the nostrils, in the form of a powder or snuff, it produces violent and repeated sneezing, with a slight degree of vertigo. The violent agitation produced in this way, together with a copious discharge from the nostrils, often relieves catarrh, headache, and incipient opthalmia or inflammation of the eyes. But habit soon blunts the sensibility of the organs, and much positive injury follows the habitual use of snuff. It has been a pop [15] ular remedy in many places for the cure of scald-head, psora, and most other cutaneous eruptions. It has also been applied for cleansing ulcers, and for the removal of indolent tumors. But the dreadful effects produced by it when absorbed into the system, have induced most medical men to abandon it altogether, and prescribe a more safe application.

Though it is said, by Dr. Brailsford, to be a *sudorific* of considerable efficacy, I am in possession of no facts which go to support such a conclusion, unless indeed it be the fact, that it in an eminent degree brings on that cold perspiration of which we have spoken, and which is, in many instances, the immediate precursor of death.

But of all others, its *diuretic* properties have been the most lauded. Dr. Fowler was the first to bring them extensively into notice. In dropsy, dysury, gravel, and nephritis calculosa or inflammation of the kidneys, the infusion and tincture were given by him with astonishing success. In spasmodic asthma, the same distinguished physician found it to afford relief.

Mr. Earle, a surgeon of some eminence, has more recently treated several inveterate cases of retention of urine on the same plan and with similar effects, and adds his testimony to its efficacy in tetanus, trismus, and other spasmodic affections. Of its power to relieve spasm there can be no doubt. What has been related of its sedative qualities, is abundantly sufficient to establish that fact. Cramps, convulsions, and even the vital principle itself, give way before the exhibition of this deadly narcotic. Hence, to its power of prostrating the muscular energy, it owes its efficacy in preventing retention of urine.

We have now gone through with an examination of the medicinal properties of tobacco, and have arrived at the following conclusion, viz. that few substances are capable of exerting effects so sudden and destructive, as this poisonous plant. Prick the skin of mouse with a needle, the point of which has been dipped in its essential oil, and immediately it swells and dies. Introduce a piece of common "twist," as large as a kidney bean, into the mouth of a robust man, unaccustomed to this weed, and soon he is affected with fainting, vertigo, nausea, vomiting, and loss of vision. At length the surface becomes deadly pale, the cold sweat gathers thick upon his brow, the pulse flutters or ceases to beat, a universal tremor comes on, with slight spasms and *other* symptoms of dissolution. As an emetic, few articles [16] can compare with it for the promptness and efficiency of its operation; at the same time there are none which produce such universal debility. As a cathartic, it produces immediate and copious evacuations, with great prostration of strength; but its dose can with difficulty be regulated.

If such be a fair statement of its effects on the human system; if it requires all the skill of the most experienced practitioner to guard against those sudden depressions which uniformly follow its use, when administered with the utmost circumspection; and if, with all this caution, its operation is still followed by the most alarming, and even fatal consequences—what shall we say of those who habitually subject their constitutions to the destructive influence of this worse than "Bohan Upas?"

To an individual unacquainted with the fact, it would seem incredible that a weed, possessed of properties so poisonous, should ever have been sought as an article of luxury. Yet it has not only been sought, but even credulity startles at the extent to which it has been used. "Like opium, it calms the agitations of our corporeal frame, and soothes the anxieties and distresses of the mind." Its powers are felt and its fascinations acknowledged, by all the intermediate grades of society, from the sot who wallows in the mire of your streets, to the clergyman who stands forth a pattern of moral excellence, and who ministers at the altar of God. For it the Arab will traverse, unwearied, his burning deserts; and the Icelander risk his life amidst perpetual snows. Its charms are experienced alike, by the savage who roams the wilds of an American forest, and the courtier who rolls in luxury and prescribes rules of refinement to the civilized world; by the miscreant who wrings from the cold hand of charity the pittance that sustains his life, and the monarch who sways his sceptre over half the globe; by him who is bent with woes and years, and him whose cheek is covered yet with boyhood's down. Hence we might conclude it capable of giving strength to the weary, vivacity to the stupid, and wisdom to men void of understanding; capable of soothing the sorrows of the afflicted, of healing the wounds of the spirit, and assuaging the anguish of a broken heart. But how it fulfils these desirable indications, will be our next business to inquire.

Tobacco, as a luxury, has been used for the two last centuries over all the civilized, and the greater portion of the [17] uncivilized world. The modes have been *snuffing, smoking,* and *chewing.* Its effects, when habitually used in each of these modes, will now be examined. As far as my observations extend, few, if any, of all the devotees to this stupefying substance, ever resort to its use without some supposed necessity; and often, alas *too often,* by the advice of physicians.

The benefit to be derived from the exhibition of a medicine in the cure of disease, should not alone induce us to prescribe it, without due regard to the injury which may result to the constitution. Had this rule been observed relative to the subject under consideration, I apprehend the use of this baneful drug would have been less extensive.

Snuff has been prescribed for a variety of complaints, among which are headache, catarrh, and some species of opthalmia, and no doubt sometimes with very good effect; as I have, in a very few instances, witnessed. But the fact seems to have been overlooked, that its only power to relieve these complaints arises from the copious discharge of mucus from the nostrils, during the violent paroxysm of sneezing which invariably attends its first application; and that its salutary influence ceases, whenever these peculiar effects cease to accompany its exhibition. Hence in all cases where it is continued an indefinite time, or until the schneiderian membrane loses its sensibility, it not only fails of its medicinal effect, but actually becomes pernicious; aggravating the very disease it was intended to cure. It not only does this, but goes on committing great ravages on the whole nervous system, superinducing hypocondria, tremors, and premature decay of all the intellectual powers. A thickening of the voice, is also the unavoidable result of habitual snuff-taking. This disagreeable consequence is produced, either by partially filling up the nasal avenues, or by destroying the sensibility of the parts. Be that as it may, we would say of the change, in the forcible language of Cowper: "O! it is fulsome, and offends me more than the nasal twang, heard at conventicle from the pent nostril, spectacle bestrid."

It also occasions loss of appetite, frequent sickness at the stomach, with many other disagreeable symptoms. A case in point, is related by Dr. Cullen, of a woman who had been in the habit for twenty years. At length she found on taking a pinch before dinner, she had no appetite. This hav [18] ing frequently occurred, she was induced to postpone her pinch till after dinner, when she ate her meal with her accustomed relish, and went on snuff-taking in the afternoon without inconvenience.

Another instance is related by the same author, of the injurious effects of this habit. A lady, who had been accustomed to take snuff freely, was seized with a severe pain in her stomach, which continued unabated notwithstanding many remedies were applied; until accidentally her snuff was omitted for a few days, when the pain was found to subside, and did not return until she again had recourse to her snuff. Then, to her utter astonishment, it immediately came with all its former severity, and would yield to no treatment without a relinquishment of the snuff-box, which (strange to tell) the woman laid aside, and recovered her health.

Most persons in the constant habit of taking snuff, are led on insensibly, until they consume enormous quantities. But as they are accustomed both to its stimulant and narcotic effects, they are not aware of the pernicious consequences. In the midst of interesting conversation, they frequently transcend the bounds assigned them by habit, and the consequence is, sickness, faintness, and trembling, with some vertigo and confusion of head. During this paroxysm of snuffing, particles of the powdered tobacco are carried back into the fauces, and thence into the stomach; which occasions not only sickness at the time, but is long after followed with dyspepsia and other symptoms of disordered abdominal viscera.

The second mode of habitually using this drug, is *smoking*. This, too, has been prescribed by reputable members of the faculty. And for what purpose has this disgusting practice been recommended? "For weakness of the stomach," to be sure. Persons who have a craving appetite, and consume more food, particularly at dinner, than their stomach will readily digest, experience considerable uneasiness for some time after eating. The mouth and fauces sympathize with the overloaded organ, and an increased quantity of fluid is poured from the mucous follicles and salivary glands, to aid in the process of digestion. Under these accumulating difficulties, the man calls on the "*Doctor*," who very wisely imagines these symptoms are sufficient evidence that he has a "weak and watery sto [19] mach," and the pipe and cigar are recommended to carry off the superabundant humors, which still are unable to assimilate the enormous load with which, from time to time, the stomach is crowded. But as the application of the burnt oil of tobacco to the mouth and fauces, from its stimulant and narcotic qualities, benumbs the senses and renders the individual less conscious of his distress, he takes it for granted that he is materially relieved, and knows not, poor man, that it is all delusion. Thus, instead of taking the only rational method, that of adapting the quantity of food to the powers of digestion, he pursues a course which continues to weaken the organs of digestion and assimilation, and at length plunges him into all the accumulated horrors of dyspepsia, with a complete prostration of the nervous system.

But it has been said, that smoking will cure the tooth-ache; and we should have recourse to any means for the removal of so painful a disease. That it will, as a powerful sedative, lessen the pain, and sometimes even altogether remove tooth-ache, is probably true; but why continue the practice after the occasion has ceased? Opium and calomel, judiciously administered, will relieve *cholera morbus*; but whoever thought of making them an article of diet, because from their application he had experienced relief in that dangerous complaint? Or whoever dreamed of using them constantly, lest he might again be attacked with it? Would not prudence dictate to lay them aside, that they might not lose their influence on the system, and consequently their medicinal virtues?

But smoking sometimes diminishes the secretions of the mouth, producing dryness and thirst, instead of moisture; still it is used with the same perseverance as in the former case, and to obviate the same difficulty, an overburdened stomach. And such is the united influence of its stimulant and narcotic qualities, that the *thirst it occasions is not to be allayed by ordinary drinks, but wine, ale, and brandy must be taken, to satisfy this unnatural demand.* Hence, smoking has, in many instances, been the sad precursor to the whiskey-jug and brandy-bottle, which together have plunged their unfortunate victims into the lowest depths of wretchedness and woe.

I am well acquainted with a man in a neighboring county, whose intellectual endowments would do honor to any station, and who has accumulated a handsome estate; but whose habits, of late, give unerring premonition to his [20] friends of a mournful result. This man informed me that it was the fatal thirst occasioned by smoking his cigar, in fashionable society, that had brought him into his present wretched and miserable condition. Without any desire for ardent spirit, he first sipped a little gin and water, to allay the disagreeable sensations brought on by smoking, as water was altogether too insipid to answer the purpose. Thus he went on from year to year, increasing his stimulus from one degree to another, until he lost all control over himself; and now he stands as a beacon, warning others to avoid the same road to destruction.

Smoking has been prescribed for spasmodic asthma, and undoubtedly with some success; and the manner in which it affords relief in this distressing disease has been pointed out, when speaking of the narcotic and antispasmodic effects of this drug. But suppose it capable of relieving the paroxysm, when administered to a person unaccustomed to its deadly stimulus, it will by no means be followed by the same happy effect, when once its use becomes habitual.

But smoking has been the grand resort to secure the system from the influence of contagion; and perhaps no power ascribed to it, has ever been so universally acknowledged. But upon what series of experiments are these pretensions founded? From all the attention which I have bestowed on this investigation, I have been unable to discover any evidence of its utility in this respect, except what arose from the prejudices of the ignorant, or the obstinacy of those who are slaves to the practice of it. The bare assertion of Deimerbroek, "that it kept off the plague," without a single corroborative fact, would hardly be sufficient authority on which to establish a conclusion so important; especially when we have the united experience of Rivernus, Chemot, and Cullen, to prove the opposite of this position. Hence we conclude, that its properties in keeping off contagion, depend on its sedative powers, which it possesses in common with other narcotics, wine, brandy, and opium. As these lessen sensibility, and sometimes allay anxiety of the mind, it is not impossible that in a very few instances they may have prevented the exciting causes of disease from taking effect. But what are these few, when compared with the multitudes whose nervous systems have been destroyed by this pernicious habit, and thus exposed to all the horrors of malignant disease.

[21]

Smoking also assuages the *tedium* of life. Here is the grand secret. Man fears to be alone; and when left to his own solitary reflections, he dreads the result of self-examination. He flies for relief to his pipe, his cigar, his quid, or his bottle, with the vain hope of escaping from himself. To accomplish an object so desirable, he hesitates not to *stupify* those noble faculties which he cannot hope to extinguish, and with which he has been endowed by the God of nature, for wise and benevolent purposes. And will you, gentlemen, by precept and example, longer sanction *such* a course of conduct, — conduct so degrading to us as intelligent beings, and as conservators of the public health?

The third mode of habitually using tobacco, is *chewing*. In this manner all its deadly powers are speedily manifest, in the commencement of the practice, as has been already shown. In this mode, too, its nauseous taste and stimulant property excite and keep up a profuse discharge from the mucous follicles and salivary glands. Probably to this circumstance alone, is owing the superior efficacy of this mode of using this drug in the cure of tooth-ache. But whether this enormous waste of the secretions of the mouth and fauces can be borne by the constitution with impunity, you, Gentlemen, are abundantly competent to judge. Physiologists agree that these secretions are intended to assist in preparing the aliments for deglutition, by rendering them sufficiently fluid, and afterwards, by their peculiar properties, to promote digestion and assimilation. The great increase of these just before and after eating, and the large quantities swallowed about that time, are unequivocal evidence of their importance to the digestive economy. Then what must be the state of that man's digestion, who, until seated at table, keeps his quid in his mouth, and immediately returns it thither, after rising from his meal? And when we reflect, that large quantities of saliva strongly impregnated with this poison, and even particles of the substance itself, are frequently swallowed, what, again I ask, is the probable condition of such a person's digestive organs?

I know it may be said in reply, that such persons often consume large quantities of food, without experiencing any perceptible inconvenience; and I also know that they are often emaciated, notwithstanding the enormous portion of aliment they daily consume. Under these circumstances [22] the emaciation arises, either from the profuse discharge of saliva, or an imperfect digestion, or the combined influence of both. Hence, when a man of a corpulent habit, with a keen appetite, who is unwilling to forego his wine and to use moderation in his roast beef, applies for professional advice to prevent corpulence, medical men very naturally and philosophically direct him, if he persists in his excess, to the use of tobacco, as a temporary relief, against the direful effects of his gluttony and intemperance.

A clergyman of high standing informed me, that he acquired the habit of using tobacco in college, and had continued the practice for a number of years; but he found, by experience, his health materially impaired, being often affected with sickness, lassitude, and faintness. His muscles also became flabby and lost their tone, and his speaking was seriously interrupted by an elongation of the uvula. His brother, an intelligent physician, advised the discontinuance of his tobacco. He laid it aside. Nature, freed from its depressing influence, soon gave signs of returning vigor. His stomach resumed its wonted tone, his muscles acquired their former elasticity, and his speaking was no more annoyed by a relaxation of them.

A respectable man of my acquaintance, about forty years of age, who commenced chewing tobacco at the age of eighteen, was for a long time annoyed by depression of spirits, which increased until it became a settled melancholy, with great emaciation, and the usual symptoms of that miserable disease. All attempts to relieve him proved unavailing, until he was persuaded to dispense with his quid. Immediately his spirits revived, his countenance lost its dejection, his flesh increased, and he soon regained his health. Another man, who used tobacco very sparingly, became affected with loss of appetite, sickness at stomach, emaciation, and melancholy. From a conviction that even the small quantity he chewed was the source of his trouble, he entirely left it off, and very soon recovered.

I was once acquainted with a learned, respectable, and intelligent physician, who informed me, that from his youth he had been accustomed to the use of this baneful plant, both by smoking and chewing. At length, after using it very freely while indisposed, he was suddenly seized with an alarming vertigo, which, without doubt, was the result of this destructive habit. This afflicting complaint was pre [23] ceded by the usual symptoms which accompany a disordered stomach, and a relaxation of nerves, with which, Gentlemen, you are too familiar to need a description here. After the application of a variety of remedies to little or no purpose, he quit the deleterious practice, and though his vertigo continued long and obstinate, he has nearly or quite recovered his former health. And he has never doubted but that the use of tobacco was the cause of all his suffering in this disagreeable disease. Many more cases might be cited, but sufficient has been said to establish the doctrine here laid down. [C]

Having gone through with an examination of the *physical* influence of tobacco, let us now, for a few moments, attend to its *political* and *moral* influence.

1. *It is a costly practice.* The whole adult population in the United States is estimated at six millions, one half of which are males. Allowing but one half of these to use tobacco in some form, we shall have one and a half millions to be taxed with this consumption. If we take into the account all who are in its use before they arrive at the period of adult age, it would swell the amount to two millions. Lest we should be accused of exaggeration, we will estimate the whole number of devotees at one million, who pay their daily homage at the shrine of this stupifying idol. The expense to the consumers of this drug varies, according to the quantity and mode of using. Those who are in the habit of smoking freely, and use none but the best Spanish cigars, pay a tax, I am informed by good judges, of not less than fifty dollars a year. While the moderate consumer of Scotch snuff pays from one to two dollars. Somewhere between these wide extremes, may be found the fair estimate of an average

cost. If one fifth of the whole number of consumers should pay the highest estimate, it would amount to ten millions annually. Then if three-fifths pay but ten dollars apiece, it will amount to six millions; and if the remaining [24] one-fifth pay but one dollar each, we shall have two hundred thousand dollars more. These added together will make an aggregate of *sixteen millions two hundred thousand dollars*. In this estimate nothing has been said of another class of consumers, which delicacy forbids me to mention, (and I hope I shall receive their forgiveness for my neglect;) nor of the time wasted in procuring and devouring this precious morsel. But lest even this very moderate calculation should be considered extravagant, which is by many competent judges believed to be far too low, we will reckon the consumers at one million, and the average cost at ten dollars each a year, for the whole; and then we have *the enormous tax of three millions of dollars*, to be annually paid in these United States for the useless consumption of this loathsome drug.

2. *This practice paves the way to drunkenness.* A few reasons have already been given, why *smoking* tends strongly to favor the introduction of ardent spirits. The dryness of mouth induced in some, is not the only case where a thirst for strong drink is produced. The great waste of saliva, occasioned both by smoking and chewing, has the same dangerous tendency. The fact that few of all the consumers of this plant are fond of those simple beverages so grateful to the unvitiated taste, and that most are inordinately attached to ale, wine, and brandy, is sufficient evidence of the dreadful truth, that it is the faithful pioneer to intemperance. What though there are some few and honorable exceptions; and what though there are *many*, who for a long time have used the poisonous plant, and have escaped the yawning gulf; still, a sufficient number have been swallowed up, to warrant the general conclusion. The few specifications already made above, might easily be increased a hundred fold.

Though every lover of tobacco is not a slave to rum, yet *almost every drunkard is a slave to tobacco*; and this is indirect evidence that the habits are in a manner associated, or have a sort of natural affinity. If such be its tendency, what moral responsibility rests upon the man who shall recommend it, either by professional advice, or by his own example! What an infinitude of moral evil *must* follow in its train, if drunkenness be its legitimate effect! What woes, what sorrows, what wounds without cause, may spring into existence at your bidding, when you prescribe the ha [25] bitual use of this baneful plant! By such a prescription you incautiously open a fountain from which may issue streams, disturbing the peace of private families, pouring the waters of contention into peaceful and harmonious neighborhoods, embittering every condition of life, and poisoning every department of human society. [D]

3. *It is an indecent practice.* To say nothing of the disagreeable contortions of countenance assumed by the great variety of snuffers, smokers, and chewers; to say nothing of the pollution, inseparable from these habits, to the mouth, breath, and apparel, to the house and its furniture, (all which are too familiar to require description;) I ask, where is the man making any pretensions to refinement, who would not blush to offend the delicate sensibilities of the *fair*, by smoking his pipe or cigar in their presence? True politeness would seem to require, moreover, that even the feelings of *gentlemen* should be respected. But all sense of propriety seems to have fled before the indulgence of this foolish habit. To such an extent has it obtained, that we meet it in the kitchen, in the dining-room, and in the parlor; in every gathering of men of business; in every party of pleasure; in our halls of legislation; in our courts of justice; and even the sanctuary of God is sometimes polluted by this loathsome practice. It is impossible to walk the street without being constantly assailed by this noxious vapor, as it is breathed from the mouths of all classes in community, from the sooty chimney-sweep, to the parson in his sacerdotal robe. You can scarcely meet a man in the street, with whom you have business, but he pours a stream of smoke into your face, exceedingly disgusting. And this he does too, without imagining that he transgresses the rules of politeness, or gives you any cause of offence.

In these habits we resemble the *Aborigines* of our country. They load their huge pipes with the dried leaves of this plant, and when lighted, they breathe the dark cloud of smoke from their mouth and nostrils, and as it curls around their head, ascending towards heaven, they present it as an offering to appease the anger of the Great Spirit. A mutual influence has resulted from our intercourse with the Indian. We have taught him how to debase himself below [26] the brute, and destroy the quiet of savage life by the use of our *whis-*

key; and he, in return, has taught us to destroy our constitutions, and interrupt the harmony of civilized society, by the habitual use of his deadly narcotic. [E]

Gentlemen, I have done. The subject, with a slight examination, is before you. I have plainly and fearlessly expressed my opinion, without intending to wound the feelings of a single individual. If your sentiments correspond with mine, you will assist in bringing this odious practice to the bar of public opinion. There let it be subjected to a severe, but dispassionate trial; and if on a cool and deliberate investigation, its pernicious tendency shall fully appear, then let the American people rise up, and with united voice pronounce its sentence of final condemnation.

Footnotes

[A] See Rees' Cyclopedia.

[B] Dictionary of Arts and Sciences.

[C] And here I am happy in having permission to give the opinion of one of the ablest physicians in Massachusetts, as to the use of tobacco. "The chewing of tobacco," says he, "is not necessary or useful *in any case that I know of*: and I have abundant evidence to satisfy me that its use may be discontinued without pernicious consequences. The common belief, that it is beneficial to the teeth, is, I apprehend, entirely erroneous. On the contrary, by poisoning and relaxing the vessels of the gums, it may impair the healthy condition of the vessels belonging to the membranes of the socket, with the condition of which, the state of the tooth is closely connected."

[D] An eminent writer in favor of Temperance, has given it as his opinion, that at least one tenth of all the drunkards were made such by the use of Tobacco.

[E] The counsel given by the Journal of Health, is, therefore, in perfect accordance with the principles of medical philosophy. "Our advice is, to desist, immediately and entirely, from the use of tobacco in every form, and in any quantity, however small."—"A reform of this, like of all evil habits, whether of smoking, chewing, drinking, and other vicious indulgences, to be efficacious, must be *entire*, *and complete*, from the very moment when the person is convinced, either by his fears or his reason, of its pernicious tendency and operation."

[27]

APPENDIX,

CONTAINING AN ANSWER TO SEVERAL QUESTIONS RELATING TO THE
USE OF TOBACCO.

"But," says the lover of tobacco, "how can it be so deleterious when multitudes, who apparently enjoy good health, use it daily?"

In this objection two things are assumed, viz.

1. The existence of a perfect standard of health.

2. That this standard is not depreciated by the habitual use of tobacco.

If we examine these positions in the light of truth, we shall find them both defective.

"The varieties in point of health," says an eminent physiologist, "are numerous and considerable. There is, indeed, a certain state of health, which may be said to be peculiar to each individual. Such persons as we suppose to be in the enjoyment of the most perfect health, differ surprisingly, not only from each other, but from their own condition at other times, as well in consequence of a difference in the constitution of the blood, as a diversity of tone and other vital energies." One state may be said to be healthy compared with another; and the same may be affirmed of persons. One may enjoy health when compared with an invalid. In all these cases it will be seen that health is only comparative. But to sustain this part of the objection it would be necessary to prove, what I presume will not be attempted, "that the thousands who daily use tobacco, are enjoying the maximum of health and strength;" i. e. that every function of the system is performed to absolute perfection. For if it be admitted that any function is deranged, it would be difficult, I apprehend, to prove, that that derangement was not occasioned by the use of tobacco.

That men accustomed to hard labor will endure more fatigue, than those of sedentary or enervated habits, needs no argument to prove. That the arm of the blacksmith acquires strength beyond the arm of the literary recluse, is altogether obvious.

The laborer will consume more food; consequently his frame will acquire a proportionate degree of strength, and, all other things being equal, it will be able to resist the influence of extraneous causes, to a much greater extent than that of the voluptuary.

[28]

Let now the blacksmith use tobacco, and although there may be no perceptible diminution of vigor, (since you have no perfect standard to try it by,) because he still exceeds in strength persons possessing constitutions naturally less vigorous, or constitutions less hardened by toil; yet, whether the same hardy son of Vulcan can endure more hardship, while using tobacco, than he could have done had he never used the baneful plant, is the question?

That many persons apparently enjoy good health, and yet use tobacco, cannot be denied. And the same may be affirmed with equal propriety of opium and alcohol. I once knew a man who, from his youth till he had reached his sixty-ninth year, became intoxicated, whenever he could procure sufficient liquor to produce this effect; and during that time he was never so ill as to require medical advice. I have known others to be literally steeped in ardent spirit, who were seldom sick; and yet few, I apprehend, will affirm, that alcohol used to such excess is not injurious.

The Turks, who, for aught to the contrary that appears in their history, enjoy as good health as the people of the United States, and are said to attain a longevity as great, use opium for the purpose of intoxication, much in the same manner in which the latter employ alcohol and wine, these being forbidden to the former by their creed. Yet, after all, the man who could adduce these facts to prove the harmlessness of the substances under consideration, must be destitute of that physiological knowledge which is necessary to understand the natural operations of the human system.

There is a principle in the animal economy, which powerfully resists morbid impressions, and tends to expel whatever is noxious. This principle, called by some "the medical power of nature," is roused to action by the application of an offending agent to any part of the human system. On the first intimation of the assault, this vigilant sentinel rallies her forces, and flies to the point of attack.

If she succeed in expelling the invader before any serious mischief has been done, the system again reposes in quiet; but if not, a more general tumult arises, and the assistance of art is often required to second her ineffectual efforts. These phenomena are exhibited in the first use of tobacco, in all its forms.

Apply snuff to the nostrils of one unaccustomed to it; and a violent sneezing, with a copious secretion of mucus will follow. Put tobacco into the mouth and it immediately produces a profuse discharge of saliva; and if this proves unsuccessful in expelling the unwelcome intruder, severe nausea and vomiting ensue. Smoking also produces similar effects. Apply the moistened leaves of tobacco to any part of the surface of the body, and its deadly effects are soon perceived in an entire prostration of strength, accompanied with ghastly paleness and vomiting.

If it were not in a high degree poisonous, no such results would follow its first application to the living fibre; for they do not follow the first application of those substances which were, by our wise and bountiful Creator, designed for the *use* of man.

Though the effects above described are less violent, when the nerves (the media through which it operates) become accustomed to the stimulus of the noxious substance; yet it by no means proves, even in these circumstances, that it does no injury to the system, any more than the fact that some men drink a quart of proof spirit daily without [29] producing death, proves that that amount does them no harm, when half the quantity taken by a beginner would prove fatal.

In the course of twelve years' observation on the effects of narcotics upon the human system, I became acquainted with a delicate female, who, for thirty years, had taken a sufficient quantity of opium daily to kill the hardiest son of New-England, provided he had been unaccustomed to its pernicious influence. She, nevertheless, lived to an advanced age, and was eighty-four years old when I last saw her, though she, at that time, took every day two scruples of solid opium.

I had the unpleasant task to attend this lady in a fit of sickness. And with the exception of a few cases, in which similar results have followed the excessive use of alcohol, it was, without exaggeration, the most troublesome case that has ever fallen under my care.

All the frightful symptoms of *delirium tremens* waited around and haunted her imagination through the day; while shrieks, and groans, and all the signs of woe attended her nightly couch, to add a gloomy horror to her unrefreshing and broken slumbers. And so far as my observations extend, the most inveterate derangements of the nervous system are either produced or aggravated by the habitual use of narcotics.

The inherent power of the constitution to sustain itself amid the ever-varying changes to which it is exposed, has been learned by common observation, as well by the peasant as by the man of erudition. The fact, that man, "made of one blood, can dwell" in all the varieties of climate, "on the face of the whole earth," and can sustain himself, without any change of organization, at one period on the burning sands of a Numidian desert, at another among the ice-bergs of a Greenland winter—exhibits in the most convincing light the extent of this wonderful power.

A curious field of speculation, on this sanative power in the physical constitution of man, lies open to out view, had we time to pursue it, in contemplating the habits, customs, and manners of the North American Indian. Guided by the simple dictates of nature, he gratifies his appetite with such food as comes most readily within his reach, and slakes his thirst at the first mountain brook. Sometimes, for days, he lies sleeping in his smoky wigwam without the means of appeasing hunger; then rises and follows his game with the fierceness of a tiger, until the object of his pursuit is overtaken; after which, with the voracity of a dog, he loads his stomach with food sufficient to satisfy the cravings of nature, for as many days as he had previously fasted, and again betakes himself to sleep and inactivity. With all this irregularity, he is a total stranger to lingering complaints, and to that numerous as well as fashionable class of diseases denominated "Nervous." That formidable ailment, *Dyspepsia*, which, like a fiend, has, for the last few years pervaded the whole land, is unknown to the Indian; having its origin in the abuses introduced by civilization and refinement. But to return:

Suppose, for the sake of argument, that a man who daily uses tobacco, enjoys equal health with one who uses none, and is no more liable to disease; let him once be attacked by disease, and then it will be far more difficult to remove it, than to do so in one free from such habit.

This will appear from the following considerations :

Remedial agents ordinarily act on the system, by exciting the liv [30] ing power through the medium of the nerves; hence when these have long been deadened by the habitual use of any narcotic, common sense, aside from the lights of science and philosophy, would teach us the difficulty of making an impression on a system whose nerves had thus been previously paralyzed.

Perhaps the man, who daily drinks ardent spirit, may, from the greater insensibility of his system, in some cases escape sickness as long as the most temperate, (though this is by no means a common fact); yet, let disease once commence, and then we learn, by painful experience, the disadvantage of having broken down the nervous system by needless and vicious excess.

Tobacco is acknowledged to be one of the most deadly of the vegetable narcotics: yet experience proves that the nerves, by habit, become so accustomed to its stimulus, that it in a great measure loses its power. How then can we hope with ordinary remedies to make an impression, when even this powerful agent has itself lost its proper and natural effect?

The unparalleled mortality of the great epidemic of 1812 and 1813, was in a good measure owing to the immense quantities of ardent spirit consumed by the victims of that fatal malady. In the town in which I then resided, about forty adults died in the course of the winter and spring; and most of those were in the habit of using ardent spirit freely. And though numbers of temperate persons were attacked, yet many of these recovered; while every instance within my knowledge, where an intemperate person was attacked with this formidable disease, it proved fatal.

The ravages of the *cholera* in India and Persia, since 1816: and in the North of Europe, for the last eighteen months; settle the point in question beyond reasonable doubt. In one hundred cases where the cholera proved fatal, ninety of them had been in the liberal use of ardent spirit. And this fact should be carefully noted, when this formidable disease has reached Great Britain, and threatens us with its visitation.

If then the habitual use of alcohol, by exhausting the nervous energy, predisposes the system to disease, and at the same time renders the disease, when it has commenced, so much more intractable; what shall be said of the common use of tobacco, which is allowed by all to be a still more deadly poison, and of course must exhaust the power of the nerves in a proportionate degree?

A female, aged 27 years, was attacked in December 1829 with a sore mouth, accompanied with diarrhœa and profuse salivation. These complaints continued to increase, notwithstanding the application of a variety of remedies, prescribed by her medical attendant, until the 5th of March following, when I was called to take charge of the patient. She was much emaciated. The discharge from the bowels continued unabated, and was often attended with severe pain and great prostration of strength. The salivation was accompanied with a burning or scalding sensation in the mouth and stomach, which proved excessively irritating to the patient, as well as perplexing to me. On examining her case, I found the nervous system entirely deranged and much broken by the habit of smoking, which she had practiced to great excess from the age of eleven years. I learned, to my surprise and regret, that she commenced this habit, which afterwards cost her [31] so much suffering, by the advice of some wise member of the Faculty, who had prescribed it for some slight derangement of the stomach.

My first efforts were directed to repair the injuries inflicted by the tobacco-pipe; and though the difficulties to be overcome were many and obstinate, by patience and perseverance they were all surmounted, and the woman was at length restored.

The conflict which this poor woman endured, in overcoming a habit that not only injured her health, but nearly destroyed her life, was dreadful beyond description. When her pain and distress were great, she would complain more of this privation, than of all her other sufferings; and so strong was the desire for smoking, that she, several times during her recovery, contrary to my orders, indulged in it a few minutes, and each time with manifest injury; so that she finally was induced to abandon it altogether, and thus recovered her health. Indeed, she now enjoys better health than she has done for years.

Any one acquainted with this ordinary effects of this foolish indulgence in the free use of narcotics, on the nervous system of its victims, will be convinced by a few years close observation, that such persons especially, if they are of sedentary habits, are more subject to fits of despondency, and to a far greater degree, than persons of the same general health and of the same employment, but who have escaped contamination.

I shall here introduce the following extract of a letter, from a respectable clergyman to the author, as illustrative of this point.

"When I say that the effects of the habitual use of tobacco on the human system, are injurious; I speak from years of painful experience. I commenced the use of tobacco when young, like many others, without any definite object, but experienced no very injurious consequences from it until I entered the ministry. Then my system began to feel its dreadful effects. My voice, appetite, and strength soon failed; and I become affected with sickness at the stomach, indigestion, emaciation, and melancholy, with a prostration of the whole nervous system. For years my health has been so much impaired as to render me almost useless in the ministry, and all this I attribute to the pernicious habit of smoking and chewing tobacco. And had I continued the practice, I doubt not but that it would have brought me to an untimely grave. I was often advised to leave it off, and made several unsuccessful attempts. At length I became fully convinced that I must quit tobacco or die. I summoned all my resolution for the fearful exigency, and after a long and desperate struggle I obtained the victory. I soon began to experience the beneficial results of my conquest. My appetite has returned; my voice grows stronger, and I am in a measure freed from that mental dejection to which I once was subject. My general health is much improved, and I feel that I am gradually recovering; though it is not to be expected

I shall ever regain what I have lost by this needless and vicious indulgence. I am satisfied that the common use of tobacco is injurious to most people, especially those of sedentary habits. On them it operates with ten-fold energy. I am acquainted with many in the ministry, who are travelling this road to the grave. I uniformly say to them: "Lay aside your pipes and tobacco, or you are undone—your labors in the ministry will soon be at an end." " [F]

[F] Another Clergyman writes as follows. "I thank God, and I thank you for your advice to abandon smoking. My strength has *doubled* since I quitted this abominable practice."

[32]

A mere hint at these evils would seem to be sufficient to awaken inquiry, among the votaries of the plant in question. I shall therefore leave it to their candid decision, after a full and free investigation enables them to arrive at a just conclusion.

The great increase of *dyspepsia* within the last twenty years, with the dark and lengthened catalogue of nervous complaints that follow in its train, is, I have no doubt, in part owing to the universal prevalence of practices, the propriety of which we are calling in question.

The misery to which the consumers of this drug are subject, when from any cause they are temporarily deprived or it, would go far to deter a reflecting man from voluntarily binding himself to this most ignominious servitude. I have known a hard laboring farmer, who would have resented the name of *slave*, as much as did the Jews, arise from his bed in the middle of the night and travel half a mile to procure a quid of tobacco, because his uneasiness was such, that he could neither sleep nor rest without it. This uneasiness is more distressing than bodily pain, and has in some instances produced an agitation of mind bordering upon distraction.

Col. Burr informed Dr. Rush, that the greatest complaints of dissatisfaction and suffering, that he heard among the soldiers who accompanied General Arnold in his march from Boston through the wilderness to Quebec, in the year 1775, arose from the want of tobacco. This was the more remarkable, as they were so destitute of provisions as to be obliged to kill and eat their dogs.

The Persians, we are informed, often expatriate themselves, when they are prohibited the use of tobacco, in order to enjoy unmolested this luxury in a foreign country. Nor are these facts incredible to those, who are familiar with the laws that regulate the animal economy.

Long and obstinate is the conflict with nature, before the taste or smell of such disgusting things as alcohol, opium, and tobacco can be endured. But when she, worn out by repeated and continued assaults, abandons her post, and gives up the dominion to the artificial appetite, the order of things is reversed, and we at last find, to our sorrow, that this unnatural appetite is vastly more ungovernable than the one implanted by our Creator for things originally pleasant and agreeable. Add to all these considerations the well attested fact, that no sensible man, who has himself used the baneful weed, ever advised his neighbor or child to follow his example, but often the contrary; and its inutility is sufficiently proved.

Having thus far endeavored to shew the futility of the objection raised against our doctrine, by the consumers of this drug; let us now, in our turn, call on them to give a good reason why so much money should be expended, and so much time wasted, as are annually squandered in the various departments of raising, preparing, and consuming this plant; and to point out, if they can, in what manner a poison so deadly acts on the healthy system without producing evil consequences.

To make out the case, it will be necessary for its advocates to prove one of the following positions; either,

1. That it produces no effect at all, and is therefore harmless; or,

2. That it produces a good effect, and is indispensable to the enjoyment of perfect health.

As this part of the enquiry is somewhat important, and since it re [33] gards the success of our principles, we will examine these positions a little in detail, to see how they are sustained by fact and experience.

If it produces no effect at all, why that universal uneasiness, amounting as we have seen in some instances almost to distraction, uniformly manifested by the consumers of this plant, when by accident they are temporarily deprived of the means of indulgence?

If tobacco produces no effect, why fly to it as a solace for every woe, as a refuge from affliction and trouble, and as a hiding-place from the tempests of misfortune?

It will not, it *cannot* be doubted, that, in its power to allay the stormy agitations of mind to which we are exposed in our voyage over the tempestuous sea of life, consists the latent excellence, the *summum bonum*, of the virtues of tobacco. This sedative power will not be questioned, by those who have ever witnessed its peculiar effects.

The medicinal effects of tobacco, as applied for the removal of corporeal disorders, are nearly or quite destroyed by habitual use; but with what success it is constantly resorted to, to allay anxiety of mind, let its votaries answer.

A medical gentleman of high standing, in an adjoining county, who has recently abandoned the common use of tobacco, informed me, that on a certain occasion his muscular and vital energies were so overcome, by chewing, that in attempting to put his horse into the stable, he was obliged to lie down until he had so far recovered his strength as to enable him to proceed to his house. Many other instances were related by the same gentleman, of its injurious effects which he had observed, both on himself and others; particularly in producing watchfulness, which it was almost impossible for the greatest degree of weariness and fatigue to overcome. Many others have frequently mentioned this fact to me, since I began to investigate this subject. Now if tobacco produces no effect, why are such results witnessed by its consumers, and why do the candid among them acknowledge that these evils arise from its use? The health of the medical gentleman above named was materially improved after laying aside tobacco; and those to whom he recommended a similar course, have experienced a like favorable result.

The second position is equally unsupported either by experience or sound reasoning; and is contrary not only to all medical authority on this subject, but against the investigations of other scientific men who have chemically examined the constituent principles of tobacco, and who have experimented largely to ascertain with precision its natural operation on the living fibre. The lower order of animals have been selected for these experiments. Given in substance to them, it has uniformly proved fatal, even in very minute doses.

When its expressed juice or essential oil has been introduced under the skin of pigeons, kittens, or rabbits, it produced violent convulsions and often instantaneous death. Does any one doubt the correctness of these experiments? He can easily satisfy himself of their accuracy, by obtaining the oil of tobacco, and applying eight or ten drops to the root of a kitten's tongue. The same deadly effects, as we have seen, uniformly attend its first application to the human system, if taken to any considerable extent. This is well understood by its consumers, who are very cautious for many weeks, and even months, how they deal with the poisonous drug.

[34]

By what transformation is a plant, so deadly in its effects when first applied to the human system, afterward converted into a harmless article of diet or luxury? No substance which God has made for the common use of man, produces similar results; and if such be the fact in relation to the article in question, in this instance at least the order of nature is reversed, so that what in its nature is poisonous, becomes by habit nutritious and salutary. If this be correct reasoning—farewell to the success of temperance efforts! For *Rum*, after all, may be *convenient* if not necessary, because its effects are not in every instance immediately fatal; and because some, by dint of habit, can sustain with slight *apparent* injury, what to others unaccustomed to it would produce instantaneous death.

The stale excuse, so often repeated by the lovers of tobacco, that they have been advised to use it by physicians, for the mitigation or removal of some bodily infirmity, may be urged with equal force and propriety by the tippler and the sot; for many, very many, have been advised by members of the Faculty, to drink the deadly draught, in some form or other, either to ease the pains of dyspepsia, to allay the horrors of *tedium vitæ*, or to drown the anguish of a guilty conscience. And may not many of these patients say to those of the Faculty, who give advice for the use of either these stimulants: "Physician, heal thyself." Alas! when will the profession be without any who use ardent spirit or Tobacco.

In concluding, permit me to address a word to professors of religion on this subject.

In whatever concerns the cause of virtue and morality, you have a deep and an abiding interest. When Intemperance spreads abroad his murky "wings with dreadful shade contiguous," and fills the land with tears of blood—you look over this frightful *aceldama* and mourn at the soul-chilling spectacle. When infidelity and licentiousness exhale their pestiferous breath, to poison the moral atmosphere and destroy the rising hope of our country, by undermining the virtue of our youth; the Christian's heart is pained, and every effort is put forth to stay the march of desolation. In short, whatever tends to increase the prevalence of vice, must be witnessed by real Christians with unfeigned regret.

"Manners," says a celebrated writer, "have an influence on morals. They are the outposts of virtue." Whoever knew a rude man completely and uniformly moral? The use of tobacco, especially smoking, is offensive to those who do not practice it.

The habit of offending the senses of our friends or even strangers, by smoking in their presence, produces a want of respect for their persons; and this disposes, however remotely, to unkind treatment towards them. Hence the Methodists interdicted the common use of tobacco with that of ardent spirit, in the infancy of their society; thereby evincing a just sense of the self-denial, decency, and universal civility required by the gospel.

It is painful to witness among Christians the utter disregard of each others feelings and the rules of propriety, which have obtained in regard to these habits. They go into a friend's house, and after enjoying the hospitality of his board, sit down to smoke their pipe or cigar in his dining-room or parlor with the greatest composure; and that too, without even condescending to enquire whether it is offensive; supposing either that the appetites and senses of others are equally [35] depraved with their own, or that politeness will prevent their raising any objection to a practice which has become nearly universal. When the enquiry is made, it is understood to be nothing more than an apology for unrestrained indulgence; and the host who should intimate that it might be offensive to some, would be looked upon as having transgressed not only the rules of modern politeness, but all the laws of hospitality.

Notwithstanding the extent to which smoking prevails, there are some in almost every family, who are affected with giddiness in the head and sickness at stomach, whenever they inhale the fumes of the pipe or cigar, particularly at or near meal time. Yet all this suffering must be endured, and the fine feelings of the family disregarded. And for what? Merely to give a Christian, and perhaps a physician or a minister of the gospel, an opportunity to gratify a vicious appetite which does him no good, and which, philosophically considered, would disgrace any man who pretends to be a gentleman.

"What reception," says Dr. Rush, "may we suppose the apostles would have met with, had they carried into the cities and houses whither they were sent, snuff-boxes, pipes, cigars, and bundles of cut, or rolls of hog or pigtail, tobacco? Such a costly and offensive apparatus for gratifying their depraved appetites would have furnished solid objections to their persons and doctrines, and would have been a just cause for the clamors and contumely, with which they were every where assailed."

And yet this very disgusting practice is considered, in these days of gospel light and civil refinement, almost as an indispensable prerequisite to fit a minister of Christ to prosecute successfully the work of a missionary in evangelizing the world. Kindly expostulate with such Christians, physicians and ministers of the gospel on the propriety of their conduct, and they meet you with a multitude of the most frivolous excuses.

One uses tobacco, as the tippler does his rum, as an antidote against a damp atmosphere. Another, to prevent the accumulation of water or bile in his stomach; and a third, as a security against the encroachment of contagious diseases.

But Howard the philanthropist assures us, that it had efficacy neither in preventing the hospital fever, nor in warding off the deadly plague. Dr. Rush says, that at Philadelphia it was equally ineffectual, in preserving its votaries from influenza and yellow fever. Excuse ourselves as we may, it is at best a disgusting habit, persisted in against the convictions of our understanding and the dictates of true politeness, and adapted only to gratify a vitiated and unnatural appetite.

It is, indeed, agreeable to observe, that the superior refinement and regard to good manners, in some parts of the old world, have at length awakened public sentiment on this subject.

We are informed by travellers, that smoking is disallowed in taverns and coffee-houses in England, and that taking snuff is becoming unfashionable and vulgar in France. How much is it to be lamented, that, while the use of tobacco is thus declining in two of the most enlightened countries in Europe, it is daily becoming more general in America! "In no one view," says Dr. Rush, "is it possible to contemplate the creature man in a more absurd and ridiculous light, than in his foolish and disgusting attachment to the poisonous weed, tobacco." Who then can witness groups of boys ten or twelve years old [36] in our streets, smoking cigars, without anticipating such a depreciation in our posterity with regard to health and character, as can scarcely be contemplated without pain and horror!

After the foregoing was in type, it was submitted to Doctor Warren, of this City, with a request that he would examine the whole, carefully, and give his opinion of it. He has kindly returned the following strong testimonial in favor of the Dissertation, which cannot but secure it a wide circulation, and the attentive perusal of every man who values health.

Dear Sir—

In compliance with your request, I have read over the pamphlet of Dr. McAllister on the use of Tobacco. Though my present occupations have prevented my doing it so carefully, as to entitle me to suggest any alteration or improvement.

The general tendency of the pamphlet is excellent: and I most cordially give my opinion in its favor: for I have often had occasion to observe the pernicious effects of the free use of tobacco. Many instances of dyspepsia have come under my notice, the origin of which was traced to the practice of *chewing*; and on the abandonment of the habit, the patients were restored to health. I have seen a number of cases of injury to the voice, from the introduction of *snuff* into the *facial sinuses*. As to *smoking*, I am well satisfied that it is calculated to cause a feverish state of the body; and in certain constitutions it weakens the membranes which line the nostrils, throat, and lungs, produces a susceptibility to colds, and even more serious affections of these parts, when it has been much employed.

From what I have seen, I have been led to believe that this article is not necessary nor useful for the preservation of health; and that it is often a cause of weakness and sickness. I am, with great respect,

Your ob't serv't,

Boston, Jan. 25, 1832.   **JOHN C. WARREN.**

Note. — Many persons have the opinion that the use of tobacco is a preventive of contagious diseases: because it has been asserted that tobacconists and others living in the midst of the effluvia of this article, are exempted from the attacks of such disorders. The practices above alluded to, have in my opinion, a contrary effect. Those who live constantly in the region of tobacco, by the effect of habit cease to be stimulated and over excited by the diffusion of its lighter particles in the air they breathe. But those who employ it, occasionally, whether in smoking, chewing or snuffing, undergo an excitement, more or less considerable; which is infallibly followed by a proportionate debility, in which state, they would be subject to the attacks of a disease they might otherwise have escaped.

J. C. W.

www.ingramcontent.com/pod-product-compliance
Lightning Source LLC
Chambersburg PA
CBHW030511220526
45464CB00006B/2746

*9 7 8 3 8 4 9 1 8 4 0 5 6 *